HOMELESS
PEOPLE
EXERCISE

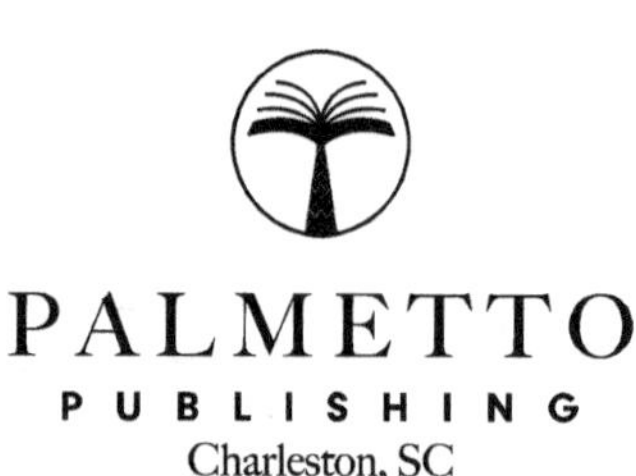

PALMETTO

PUBLISHING
Charleston, SC
www.PalmettoPublishing.com

Paperback ISBN: 979-8-8229-4287-5

HOMELESS PEOPLE EXERCISE

ALI. M.

DISCLAIMER

This booklet is intended for the purpose of the information only, and all the information presented in it, expressed solely by the author personal knowledge, and experience to share it with the public, and did not based on any medical or scientific research, and the public have the right of the option, and the full responsibility on whether to use the information in it or not, and most importantly and for the confirmation, this booklet is not intended to provide any type of medical treatment and medical consultation nor to replace any type of medical treatment and medical consultation, and it is recommended and always to seek a consultation with your medical professional or somebody professional in the field prior to conduct the exercise.

TABLE OF CONTENTS

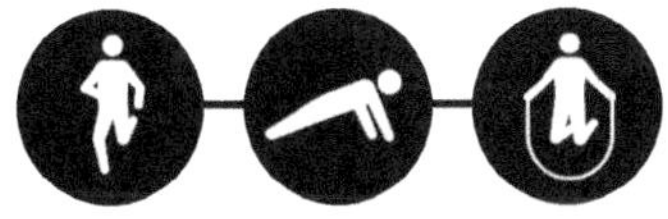

CHAPTER 1-A

Growing up in a great family, and surrounded with a great friends, whose were passionate, and filled with positive goals, and dreams in life, about becoming successful, and accomplishing great things in so many different aspects in life, and knowing that the sky has no limit, it was a very challenging and sacred responsibility, that was requiring a longevity, and lot of time, and efforts to achieve it, and it cannot be achieved from nothing, as matter of fact, by **applying, practicing and maintaining a healthy life habits, were one of these efforts that would help to achieve these positive goals**, and dreams in life.

In early childhood, particularly when I was 6 years old and before I went to the elementary school, I was advised, and taught around the clock, by my family in order to achieve all the positive goals, and dreams that I need in life, **I will need to stay in a better healthy condition both physically, and mentally for long run**, and this can be done by applying a healthy habits in my life, and one of these healthy habits, is that I need to **keep my body always** active, and there are many steps to do that, and one of these steps, was by **applying certain types of sports** into my life that I am really like and passion about it.

Once I made it in the elementary school, **that lasted 6 years**, there was a Sport Class, which was equivalent to a Fitness Class, and the Sport Class was the same importance as the rest of the other classes, however the Sport class was mandated by the school management , that all the school students need to attended and participated in it, and it was giving in the morning as first class, and mostly was about conducting some type of physical exercises such as stretching, warming, and cool down exercises, in addition to that, a running, sprinting, jogging exercises, and sometimes playing sports such as soccer, and basketball games, and the main idea behind it, was to keep the students active and healthy in both physical, and mental aspects.

Then at adolescent age, I realized that my passion, and obsession about applying, and practicing different sports, and physical exercises into my life was drastically increased, and I was excited about it, and I was expected to see all of that from happening once I made it to the Intermediate school, however at the Intermediate school that **last 3 years**, unfortunately, I was shocked there, due to the fact, that the physical exercises were giving to me in the Sport class, were similar to the physical exercises that I was learned when I was in elementary school as a result of that, I was getting bored from doing the same physical exercises, despite the fact, it was nothing wrong with it, however it was not meeting my personal expectations, in addition to that, in general, changing, and trying new aspects in life are very important, and that meant a lot for me, and for that reason, I decided to do something different than what I learned in elementary and Intermediate school. I signed up with a local Greco-Roman wrestling club after school time, and it was at my own expenses, and my family supported me with that, and my goal from that, as it was mentioned earlier which was to do something different, and also, to learn, and train, and accommodate my body into different training exercises, and the most important, was to stay healthy in both aspects physically, and mentally.

At the local club of Greco-Roman Wrestling, I was myself, with another 15 teammates of different gender, and different ages, and the majority of them, are not a professional wrestlers, as matter of fact, they were normal people with different professions, however their main goals were similar to my goal which was to learn different sports, and the most important to stay in better healthy conditions in both aspects physically, and mentally.

Inside the club, we were taught, and trained by a professional a Greco-Roman coaches, who used be a former wrestlers, and since we were in a big group, and our goals, were similar, and based on all of that, our coaches created a certain weekly **training calendar** that suit the entire groups and it won't conflict with our daily responsibilities.

The weekly training calendar consisted of two hours long a day to give everyone the opportunity to learn and understand the training, however the training was **every other day**, and in **the evening time**. So the first half hour of these two hours, was consisted of mix of certain training exercises that focused mostly on cardio, and strength, and it did not last more than a 25-30 minutes, however per the coaches guidance, these durations were varies, were sometimes it will get longer, and sometimes it will get shorter, while the rest of the time, was mostly focused on providing an educational information about rules and regulation of wrestling, and entire its techniques, and hands on by sparing within the teammates.

As far as the reason behind why my training exercises was every other day, and according to the coaches, this was related to **three factors**, and **the first factor** was that since the training exercises was consisted of cardio, and strength that required a lot of body movement, therefore it was very necessary to give the body enough time for recovery and to consume enough nutrition that would help to boost the energy, and replenish whatever lost from the training, and **the second factor,** was to give the trainees the opportunity to take care of their life responsibilities, and to balance the time between these responsibilities, and time of training, and the third factor was, since that the intention from the training exercises, was to stay in better healthy conditions, and to avoid the injuries, and that was the most important ones.

while as far as the nutrition, and due to the high cost of the sport nutrition, and supplements that were on the markets, the coaches were very considerate about that, and for the economic benefits of all the trainees, they didn't put a restrict diet or nutrition that need to be followed, therefore their best recommendation was to stay hydrated, and to enjoy whatever diet want to follow, however it has to be done with precautions in regard to the health condition, and the age group per every trainee.

As a result of the coaches' guidance, the every other day training exercises were very suitable and helpful to all to the trainees, and the outcomes of it, were very noticeable, and impressive within few weeks of the training, and this was, unlike what as usually common for some people who trained for 6 days in row in a week for certain hours with 1 day for recovery or some others trained for 5 or 4 days in-rows with certain hours too, and take 2 or 3 days for recovery, and there was nothing wrong with these calendar training exercises, because it was all dependent on the type of workout, and the intention behind it.

Despite the fact, my goal was from learning, and exercising about the Greco-Roman wrestling, was to keep my body in better health condition, I was fortunate to take parts in several Greco-Roman competitions, within some local clubs' teams, and around the country too.

Meanwhile my personal knowledge, and academic experience about applying healthy habits in my life, were improving constantly because I was reading about it, and learning about it from variant sources.

Once I made it to the high school **that last 3 years** too, I continued with Greo-Roman wrestling sport after school, however my professional experience about it, was professionally improving, moreover my fitness level was improving too, and at the same time, and per my coaches' guidance, I always kept myself hydrated, and my nutrition was not that different from what my family used to consume on daily basis, as matter of fact, I was very rare to make some modifications to my nutrition, and as we know that everybody is reacted, and responded to certain things differently than the others, therefore I felt that my nutrition was great enough for me, to **boost my**

energy for training, and to replenish whatever calories I lost from practicing a Greo-Roman wrestling.

Later, and once I made it to university, it was a shifting point in my physical fitness, were I had to quit a Greco-Roman wrestling sport, and focused **on body building sport under coach supervision**, and the reason behind that, was the same reason that I made it when I went to intermediate school, and high school with the same goals too.

Since my last experience with Greco-Roman wrestling's **weekly training calendar** was very beneficial to me, therefore I was able to apply the same weekly training calendar that was every other day, and in **the evening time too**, and my coach was fine with it, since the outcomes were positive on me both physically, and mentally, however the **duration of this body building training was only for 1 hour long**, and it was different than what it was in the Greco-Roman Wrestling training, and it was consisted mostly from weights lifting exercises, and cardio in certain days, while my nutrition continued to be the similar to what I was doing it with Greco-Roman wrestling training except in some cases, when I was feeling hungry, I had to add an extra meal to my regular daily meal, that was consisted of three meals a day, and the most important in that, that I always kept myself hydrated. I continued doing the body building training until I moved to United States.

Moving to United States, was 360 degrees shifting point in different avenues in my life, and the reason was because the available opportunities, and the freedom to change, and be something from nothing was incredibly limitless-

Despite that, the focus here in this book, will be about progression of my physical fitness, and variety of the professional knowledge that I gained from learning, and practicing different types of sports, and the most important, was in how to stay in better health condition both physically, and mentally for long run, therefore the explanation in this book will be only focusing on this topic.

In United States, the magnificent opportunities, and the availabilities of the most sophisticated information, and technologies in the field of fitness and sports, were tremendously developing, and improvising constantly, nevertheless the best academic, and training institutions in the world, and best athletes too.

However, moving into United States, and starting a new life was very challenging in variant aspects, however it was not impossible, but it was requiring an incredible dedication, focusing, and patience, to establish this new life, and for a person like me, whose new, and alone to this new life, and He was still trying his best to figure everything out there, **budgeting and saving** were one of my main priorities that I applied into my new life, in order to keep me survived there, in addition to that, the cost of living, the medical expenses, and so on, were not that easy to get it afforded, therefore survivability and establishing the foundation of the new life that I wanted to started there, were another important priorities for me , and for that reason, I worked three different jobs a week, and without any day off, and due to that, I was not able to practice nor to attend any fitness center to conducted my physical training that I used to doing it prior to my arrival to United Stated, and not even to explored it, and I decided to postponed it that until I become happily capable to afforded, that being said, my goal about staying in better healthy condition for long run didn't stop at all as matter of fact, since I was do-ing three different jobs a week, and luckily, all the three jobs were physically demanding, therefore **my body was always active, and my mind was very positive about it**, and I realized, it was a great replacement to my physical training, since it was giving me the same benefits that my body, and mind used to get from training at the fitness facility which is to stay healthy, and in good condition, while my nutrition stayed regular, and I was eating whatever I want, however I was careful on some meals for the benefit of my wellness, and hydration was very important for me, so I always stayed hydrated, and managed as well to get enough resting and enough sleep because these two are very important too, and I continued doing that for a long while.

After living for a while in United States, I started a new stage of my new life, were I quit one of three jobs that I had so that I can have more time to know, learn, and understand about my new life, and I was able to make a great friends, and figured some places out, and one of these places, was the public park, and since it was a free, I took advantage of that, and this time, I started conducting my physical training down there, however due to my new life responsibilities, and the two jobs that I had, I adjusted my physical training according to my daily routine, and to the opening, and closing hours for the public park, were I trained for **not more than 35 minutes long**, with variant times, and dates, and mostly was in the evening time, and before the sun goes down, and the park closed. I was training there for at least **2 to 3 times** a week, in addition to that, I ensured to have a good recovery time within these training days.

My training was consisted of a mixture of training exercises, that mostly was a cardio exercises such as **running**, and **walking** exercises, and some strength exercises that involved a **body weight exercises or what it called a Calisthenics**, and mostly was such as push-ups, and sit-ups in addition to that, an air body squat.

In the park, there were a free equipment exercises that were already set there, for public usage, such as the pull ups bars, and dips bars, and those helped me a lot in my training after I integrated them into it, and I was rotating between these exercises, and while my nutrition and hydration continued the same.

Few months later, I continued training over the public park, meantime, I have two friends of mine, who were having a medical conditions for not exercising their bodies for a long time, and I was approved by two of them, to speak about their stories here in my book for the purpose of benefiting from other experiences, however due to their confidently, and upon their personal request, I was not able to mentioned their names.

So both my two friend were in their middle ages, they were already have their own families, and all they cared about it, was on working hard to afford a survivability to their families, and taking care of the essential expenses only, and the coincidence that the two of them, were doing a jobs that doesn't require so much physical activities, and for over 10 hours a day for each one of them, despite to that, their jobs' pensions were barely enough to keep their families surviving from month to month, and they were fallen under a category of low class family or a family with low income, and due to that, they have not been exercising at all nor they have never been in any fitness center, and their nutrition was not watchful, because their main priorities were to keep their families surviving and being exercising, and following special nutrition for the two of them, was firstly a waste of money, since they works with minimum wages, and they can't afford that, and secondly was waste of time for the two of them, since they want to be around their families after long hours of daily working, and since they have not been doing exercising for these two, unfortunately, the two of them, were suffering from a chronic medical conditions and despite the medical professional's instruction to them to exercising for health benefits, they were still not able to do it, and based on them, the main reason that was preventing them from doing it was financial difficulties.

I was feeling sad about them, therefore I decided to help them in that, and I approached them, and explained to them the health benefits from exercising in a very simplified, and motivating ways, and the positive outcomes that their bodies will have in both aspects physically, and mentally once they started exercising, and since their budgets were the main issue that were preventing them from exercising, and in somehow, their issue was similar to my issue, and for that reason, I recommended to them to exercising the same way that I was exercising over the public park, which was not going to cost them anything, however they will need to allocated some time, and efforts from their daily routine for that, as a result of that, my two friends were not happy to give up some of their times, and life responsibilities for exercising , despite to that, I kept pushing this matter on them, and told them, that they will not lose anything, and all they need to do, is to give it a try, and later on, they can decided whether the exercising is good for them or not, and the two of them were convinced about it, and since they have not been exercising at all, therefore the three of us, agreed to meet up over the same park that I used for training for the purpose of the explanation, and to show them the techniques, I was conducting for my physical training, and type of exercises that I was using it, and the benefits for each exercise, and also, it was in very simplified and motivated matter to give them the push start, as a result of that, the two of them were very eager for it, and due to their medical conditions, I was not able to give them the same exercises that I was using in my physical train-ing, and instead of that, I recommended to them, one a simple exercise however it was a very powerful one, and that exercise was the **walking exercise**, and since they were just getting started, and due to their life respon-sibilities, I recommended to them to do **only 20 -30 minutes of walking on their own pace for every three days a week** at any place where they find it a suitable, and safe for them to conduct the exercise, and the public park was an example of many other places, and the reason was behind to do the three days of training a week, was to keep them always motivated to the training, and not to make them feel the training is becoming bored nor not to cause any negative impact on their other daily life particularly spending time with their families, and the most important to have a good recovery time.

Then I informed them, that once their bodies started getting used to the **20-30 minutes of walking**, or whatever they are started feeling that they are becoming comfortable to go more with the duration of walking, then they increase the **20- 30 minutes to 35- 45 minutes** or an **hour** with increasing their pace proregression too, and also, the frequency of the exercise can be **reduce to every two days** a week, **instead of every three days a week**, however they need to take their necessary precautions during their exercising, and also, to be very watchful to where they are stepping into it, and also to avoid over walking, because the fact, that walking is very low impact exercise with little risk involved, however injuries can still occur, beside continued over doing it, can increase the risk of injuries, soreness and burnout can occur too, in addition to that, I showed them some simple **warm up and cool down exercises** that they need to conducted prior and after to their walking, **with affordable and comfortable shoes** to wear while exercising, and as far as their nutrition, I recommended to them, to eat whatever they like to eat, however they need to be careful regarding their age, and their medical conditions, and I ensured to them, that hydration is very important, and the two of them were very positively recipient to all of that,

After few days, all the three of us, agreed to conducted the exercise together so that, they can have a full understanding of it under my watch, and after that, they were on their owns, however we stayed in contact, and within few months, the results were greatly impressive in both aspects physically, and mentally, and based on my two friends' feedback, they felt more healthier than ever despite their medical conditions, that started getting more under controlled, and their medical professionals were very impressed with that, and they encouraged them to continued exercising.

Meanwhile, I continued doing my exercise over the public park, and one of the evening time, while I was training there, I've noticed there was a group of five men of different group ages were youngest one seems in his late 40s, and the oldest ones was in his early 70s, and they seems new to the park, however they were always hung out together at the sitting benches in the park for chitchatting, and resting, and they were minding their own business, and from where they were sitting at, in small distance, I was exercising at, and this group of five men continued coming back to the park very frequently, and they were staying together in the same place, and every time I was there for training, they were there too, however this group of five men were not there when the park was closed for any reason, and from the way, this group was dressing up, and the personal belongings that have on them, those people were a homeless people, and despite to that, they were in **fine shape**, were the majority of them, **were not underweight nor overweight**, and they were in between the two, and I was wondering about it, and because of that, one day, I approached them, and introduced myself to them after greeted them, and without any hesitation, they have been done the same thing with me, then I asked them politely, about the reason why they were in a fine shape despite their socioeconomic situation, as result of that, everyone laughed and

I was surprised from that, then one of them, named was Harry, and Harry was the oldest ones in the group, and He said to me literally these words

"Hey, young man, we have been watching you while you are training, and we don't do what you are doing " as a result of that, I became more curious about what Harry told me, and I asked him about himself and the other men about what they do for training if they were not doing what I was doing, and again, everyone laughed including Harry himself, and again, I was surprised from their reaction, then Harry spoken to me, his unforgotten words

"Young man, neither me nor my buddies that you see here, are trained for nothing , as matter of fact, we are a homeless people, and each one of us, have been living in the streets, around the bus stops, the dumpsters, for some quite of years, and we do not eat as you or normal people eats because we survived on whatever help, and donation we get from the people, and we might seems to you, that we are in a fine shape, but we are not because all of us are filled with a lot of medical conditions, and the youngest one of us is 49 years old, but I know what are trying to get from your question, and I will tell you simply, we are on our feet all day, and night long, and most of the time, our feet is our only way of transportation from one place to another, and each one of us, walk 5 miles to 10 miles at least a day, and imagine doing that constantly every single day, and for quiet of years, and for that reason we seem in fine shape for you, and myself, and my buddies took that as a complement from you, and I am sure for the fact, that you, and everyone knows, in general, walking is a great exercise for the body, and being a homeless, and as I mentioned earlier that we don't train but I consider walking is **the only exercise that the vast majority of homeless people like us can afforded at no cost of any given time, and place, it is a homeless people exercise"**

As a result of that, I concluded that Harry's words were another fact for me , that walking is a great exercise for the body regardless , and everyone in our entire universe can achieve it at any given time, and place with zero cost, and I thanked Harry for his words, and ever since I became a friend with him, and his group, and every time, I was at the park for training, Harry, and his group were very courteous, and respectful to me, and to my training and never interrupted me, and I exchanged the same behavior with them, and basically, our friendship was based on mutual respect, and we kept it into this level, and every time, I was at the park, they were always greeted me by saying these words-

"A homeless people exercise or HPE" and I was responding back to them with same greeting, and ever since, these words became our greeting words, and one time, I told them, that one day, once my living condition, will changed, and become better, I am going to write a book about walking exercise, and I will name it with these greeting words, for honoring and memorizing their friendship, and they were greatly happily about that.

A year passed by, and one day, and as usual I came to the park for training, and neither Harry nor his group was there, and I was surprised from that because they were always there, and somehow, they become part of my training, were I was doing the first thing upon my arrival to the park, and prior to start my training, was to exchange greeting with them, and mind our business, and before I departed the park, I wished them a great day until my next training.

So on the next time when I came back to the park for training, neither Harry nor his group were at the park, and I felt there was something wrong with that, and because of that, I asked the park's security personal about them, and the security personal, informed me, that Harry, and his group was told to leave the park, and not to come back for some hygiene matters, and I was feeling sad about that, because I was not able to have the opportunity to say good bye to them or at least knowing to where is their next destination is going to be at after the park, despite all this time, that I knew Harry and his group, out of the respect and courtesy to them, I was never asked them about their life's back ground, and why they ended up to be a homeless, because I've noticed on them, that they had been through a lot in their life's, and I was very considerate about it, and ever since they were gone, every time I was coming to the park, and before I started my training, I was always looking at the same benching seats that Harry, and his group used to sit on it, hoping that I was see them back, unfortunately, they were never come back, and that led me to made the self-determination, to write the book that I promise them about it.

After that, life moved on, and few years later, I was fortunate take advantage of whatever opportunity was available for me, that would allow me to improve, and advance in my fitness level, and the most important expanding my professional knowledge both academically, and personally. I studied, and practiced, and become certified from different institutions, and organization around the stateside, that were focused specifically on sports, fitness, health, and nutrition, and I was able to integrate all of that into my daily life routine to establish a healthy life habits, and the most important, I was able to use what I learnt and experienced in that field for assisting, guiding, and instructing a lot of people whose their goals were to be healthier in both aspects physically and mentally to achieve the good wellness for long run to enjoy life to the fullest, in returned, the outcomes were tremendously amazing, and I was feeling very happy about it, and eager to continue doing it, and to make the world that we are living in it, a better place, because every human in this life needs to activate their roles and to use whatever specialty they have for the benefits of the others, because these are noble, and virtue things in life.

CHAPTER 1-B

As we know that, life and death are part of each other, and there is no doubt about it, and this God's matter related, however human nature love to live longer as much as the time allow them to enjoy the life to the fullest and in order to do that, there are plenty of important factors that will need to be done in the life, and one of these important factors, **is by having a good wellness for long run, and good wellness for long run can be achieved via applying a multiple healthy life habits or health program to the life, and this can be started firstly with the most important healthy habit is by exercising regularly through practicing and maintaining a**

better physical, and healthy mental habits, and these considered the foundation, and the core of good wellness, and secondly by consuming a good nutrition, and so on.

The relation within these multiple habits is correlated, and for example consuming healthy food, and exercising periodically, the outcomes will be greatly positive on the body, in both aspects physically, and mentally, and continue to do that, it will generate healthier body, and healthier mind, and vice versa.

To conducted and maintain all these healthy life habits, it might sound easy and not impossible but the reality, it might become very difficult, for some people **with middle income** to afforded, and sometimes it might get very difficult too for some people **with high income** to maintained it, or it might neither get afforded nor maintained for some people **with low income or people within the poverty line or below it**, and this is due to the fact, that life nowadays, and everything in it, it is becoming more challenging on daily basis, and **the cost of living condition** is on constant rising in every single day, and **the responsibilities that fall** on everyone it increased periodically, and this lead to distract the focus on conducting, and maintaining these healthy habits in the life.

Despite these difficulties, these healthy life habits can be achieved and maintained on regular basis, without leaving life responsibilities behind, and also, it can be achieved simply at no given cost, and place, furthermore, it does not require any type of equipment except it require a self-dedication, and self-motivation to make it happen, and the most important, it will benefits people **with different socioeconomic status** particularly the people **with low or below the poverty line**.

As it was stated earlier in chapter 1-A, that applying, practicing, and maintaining healthy life habits are very important for our life, and being in better physical, and healthy mental habits on regular basis, are one of the most important healthy life habits that need to be established in our life to accomplish whatever positive goals, and dreams in life, and to enjoy the life to the fullest.

Therefore, for the health benefits of the others, I planned, and recommended a simple, and powerful exercise that can be achieve at any given time, and place with no cost, and that is the **Walking Exercise** or as

Harry named it a **Homeless People Exercise or (HPE)**, and I decided to write a book about it in very simplified and easy platform and straight to the point, and away from any confusion, and complications, to suit everybody and everybody can benefit from it.

HISTORY OF WALKING

The history of walking has been going over a long time, and the estimate was around millions of years ago and was in Africa. As the human evolved, the walking patterns have been developed, and the Bipedalism or the walking on two legs, did not come over a night, as matter of fact, it is a history of millions of years of long walking process, and not an invention, and our ancient ancestors like hominids could walk on two legs, therefore a Bipedalism, it is an important feature that distinguished between the modern humans, and their ancestors from their predecessors.

After that, walking becomes the basic human gait for all the people, and the main source of their movement from one place to another and it does not require much energy as other forms of transportation such as vehicles or trains, and walking upright provide multiple benefits as well, it provides the human to use their free hands for carrying items, and their children while they are walking.

Walking is a common form of locomotion among legged animals including humans, and most of the time defined as series of following steps performed at least when one foot placed on the ground at any given time.

Due to the tremendous amounts of health benefits that can be offered from walking, such as burning body fat, toning muscles, and treating many diseases, and some psychological problems, it become a form of great physical exercise that everyone can achieve it at any age, as a result of that it becomes as a sport, and was introduced into the Olympic games as a race walking, and one of the traditional, and earliest method of walking was Heel to Toe Stride that involve placing the heel of the foot on the ground first followed by the ball of the foot and the toes, and within the time, walking developed, and different type of forms of walking emerged depending on the goal and terrain such as Leisure walking, that was suitable for anyone wants to walks for fun, and Nordic walking that involved a poles similar to the ski-poles while walking, and so many other forms.

Nowadays, and many countries around the world, started marketing, and urging people for walking due to the great health benefits from exercising it, and started allocated a special day for walking events, and some countries, they announced these walking events as national events in their monthly, and annual calendars.

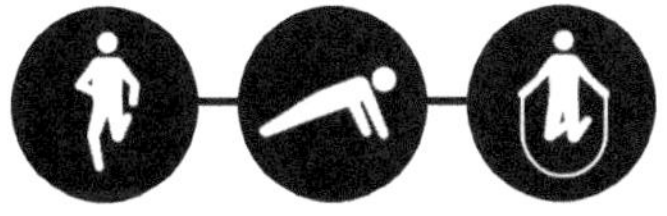

TYPES

This homeless People Exercise (HPE) is targeting people from all ages with different life categories, particularly for some whose never been exercising, or some is willing to exercise but they cannot afford it to do it for some socioeconomic reasons or some they can afford to exercise but they do not have time to attend any physical fitness facility or a senior people or some their medical conditions prevented them from practicing any type of exercise such as joints problems , and some other health problems.

This Homeless People Exercise (HPE) intend to keep us in healthier conditions, and not to make us the best athletics in the world, and maintaining a healthier conditions, it will give us the opportunity to live longer, and allow us to practice our daily life activities and enjoy it to the fullest and accomplish our dreams.

For the health benefits of everybody, and to ensure that everybody full understanding the information in this booklet and without any complications, to execute this exercise without the need of any assistance, I wrote this booklet in very simplified matter.

Walking is the one of the easiest, and the most efficient exercise that be done for the health, and it doesn't require any equipment and can be achieved anywhere, at any given time with no cost, and walking is very low impact aerobic exercise, and it is an suitable training exercise for all ages particularly elderly people, and the positive health outcomes from doing it, are tremendously amazing.

Walking is part of the human daily physical activities, and we as human our walking modes are completely different from one to another, but in general most of the human intended to walk shortly with regular pace or own pace, while they conducted their daily life activities, and sometimes, and depending on the purposes, their walking mode changed from short walk and regular pace to long walk with faster pace, and vice versa, and nothing wrong with either two, because the two of them, have a great health benefits for the body, therefore and as it was stated earlier that Homeless People Exercise (HPE) intention is to keep you healthier, and for that reason, I planned to have this exercise to be done in two types and either two are very beneficial for the body in both aspect physical, and mental, and the first type of this Homeless People Exercise, is the **Homeless People Short Walk Exercise, and the second type of it, is the Homeless People Long Walk Exercise**, and both can be done at any given time, and place, and before we execute these two exercises, there are few things that will need to be executed in order to get the best results out of these two types, and to avoid injuries, and these are the **walking posture** technique while we conducted either one of these two types, and also, some **warm up, and cool down** exercises, and some **safety** procedures.

POSTURE TECHNIQUES

When practicing the Homeless People Exercise (HPE), it is very important to know that every muscle in the body should be synchronized with each other to avoid any injuries to these muscles, and to achieve the best results of the exercise in very safe matter, and here are some posture techniques that need to be applied while conducting the Homeless People Exercise (HPE):

1. Keep your eyes forward while walking, and this can be done by keeping the head forward comfortably, and it will help you to maintain your balance, and also allowing you to watch your steps, and your path.

2. Bring both of your shoulders back, and ensured they relaxed too, however don't exaggerated about it, and at the same time, stand tall or imagine that you are a tall person, and by doing all of these, it will give you a good support to the upper body while walking and it will lower the risk for long term injury.

3. Keep the back straight, and this will not just help you to straighten your back, but also to make you breathe better while walking, due to the fact that leaning the back whether forward or backward while walking could cause neck, shoulder, and back issues such as pain, and stiffness, and sometimes muscle stiffness in long run.

4. Activate your muscle core in the abdomen, in way that keeps you comfortable, and not overreacted and this can be done by pulling in your abdomen, in other words, it's like flattening your stomach, and doing that, it will support your back while walking, and maintain the proper posture.

5. Maintain slight natural arms swings, with slight elbow bending, and this will help you to push forward.

6. Keep the natural space between your legs and your feet and this should be in line with your hips while walking, and always roll from the heel to the toe, and ensure natural, and smooth steps, or whatever make you comfortable about it.

7. Regardless of what type of walking exercise is used, always start with gradual pace then you can increase your pace or whatever makes you feel comfortable.

8. Footwear ensures to have for yourself, an affordable footwear, that can help you to walk comfortably, and also to provide enough support and protection while walking, and as far as the clothes, wear affordable sweat resistant clothes or whatever make you feels comfortable, however ensured, they are suitable for the weather, and terrains.

9. Hydration: In General, hydration is very important, therefore it is very important to keep your body hydrated at all the time, and this is doesn't matter whether you are exercising in hot or cold weathers.

WARM UP, AND COOL DOWN EXERCISES

WARM UP EXERCISE:

The primary idea from conducting the warm up exercises , are helping to preparing the body for the exercise by raising the body temperature, and the blood flow too, and this will enable to pump more oxygen to reach to the muscles in the body, as a result of that, it will minimized the risk of the injury, therefore these exercises are very important, and they need be done prior start the walking, and they should be done in 5-10 mins, and anywhere.

1. Neck rotation: Gently rotate your neck to the left and right sides for 3 times, and vice versa.

2. Shoulder rotation: Gently rotate your shoulders to the front, and rear sides for 3 times, and vice versa.

3. Arm rotation: extend your arm fully straight then gently rotate to the front, and rear sides for 3 times each, and vice versa.

4. Overhead arm clap: Gently doing it for 10 times.

5. Hand rotation: Gently rotate the hand from the wrist area to the left, and right sides for 3 times for each hand, and vice versa.

6. Hip rotation: placing your hands on the side of the hip, and gently rotated to the left, and right sides for 3 times, and vice versa.

7. Knee raise: Gently raise each knee up and down direction, for 3 times, and vice versa, and the knee

raise should be within the hip level or whatever make you comfortable.

8. Knees rotation: Brings the knees next to each other, and place the hands on them, while doing that, gently rotate them for 3 times clockwise, and 3 times counterclockwise.

9. Foot rotation: Gently rotate each foot from the ankle area for 3 times clockwise, and 3 times counterclockwise.

10. Jump exercise: Gently jump on both of your feet, as much as you can or whatever makes you feel comfortable, and you can do that for 3-5 times.

11. Air body squats: Gently do it for 3-5 times.

12. If you have any medical or physical issues that prevent you from doing some or all of these warmup exercises that mentioned above, then choose from them whatever makes you feel comfortable to do it, and you can integrate it with some of these

alternative exercises such as walking slowly in small distance for 1-2minutes, or jogging in your place for 1-2 minutes, and steps exercise or stairs exercise by simulating like you are walking up, and down the stairs, and do it gently for 1-2 minutes, and example for that, you use the side curb or small box or small chair. Lastly if you are already familiar with some warmup exercises, and you feel it can warm up your body for the exercise then by all means do it.

COOL DOWN EXERCISES:

The primary idea from conducting the cool down exercises, are helping to prepare the body to release all the muscle tension that resulted from walking, to return to its natural status prior to start the walking, and these can be done anywhere, and doesn't need more than 5 minutes to executed, and here are these cool down exercises:

1. Arm extension upper stretching pause: From a natural stance position, gently extended both arms fully straight together above the head, by holding hands together with interlaced fingers, and the palm of both hands should be faced up, and from that

position, moved the arms little pit behind the head, and paused while gently stretched there for 10 seconds, and you should feel the stretch in entire arms, and upper part of the body then release both arms to the natural position, and doing that will help to release muscles tension from upper body.

2. Deltoid cross arm extension stretching pause : From a natural stance position, start with the left arm first by crossing it fully straight on the chest area on the front toward the right side it, and keep it on the shoulder level, while the right arm placed it on the elbow of the crossing left arm- -and gently you pushed toward the upper part of chest, and paused while gently stretched there for 10 seconds, and you should feel relief in the deltoid muscle of the crossing left arm, and with right arm, and repeat the same drill, and the pause while stretching it for 10 seconds too, then release both arms to the natural position.

3. Arms extension rear stretching pause: From a natural stance position, however the feet should be little wider open, and pointed to outside, and from

there push both arms behind your back, while they are fully extended straight, and holding each other with interlaced fingers, and hand palms faced outside, and paused there while gently stretched for 10 seconds, then release both arms by returning to the natural position.

4. Glutes, Hamstring, and Calfs stretching pause: From a natural stance position, move the left leg forward in small distance with your body leaning on it, and paused while both hands placed over the hamstring of the left leg, and at the same time, move the right leg backward in small distance too, and paused, and stretched it there for 10 seconds, you will feel the release of muscle tension in your glute, hamstrings, and calf of the entire right leg, and then rotate with right leg, and repeat the same drill, then return to the natural position.

SAFETY PROCEDURES

The Homeless People Exercise (HPE) can be conducted outdoor, and indoor, and to get the best results out of it, there are a safety procedures that need to be followed, and these depend on whether the exercise was conducted outdoor, or indoor.

OUTDOOR SAFETY PROCEDURES:

These applies when the walk is being conducted outdoor such as in the public parks or around your neighborhood or in the backyard of your house or around the beach area or any open areas, and so on, and these outdoor safety procedures as follows:

1. Pathway, and Terrains: Be familiar with the pathway, and terrains, that you are planning to use for exercise, and ensure, it is intact to avoid any injuries while exercising, and safe as well as.

2. Affordable Attire: It doesn't matter whether you are walking in the sunny day or rainy day or any type of weather as long as you are prepared your body for it by wearing the proper attires (top, bottom, footwear, and wear a sleeve if you are in need for it such as knee sleeves, calf sleeves and so on), that will give you the support, and protection, and make you more comfortable while walking, and don't forget to check the forecast ahead.

3. Reflective Identification: Homeless People Exercise can be conducted at any time, however If you are planning to be exercising in the early morning or evening time or nighttime, and you think there is poor visibility, and for your personal safety ensure to wear something reflective on you to identify you such as a reflective belt or a headlamp and so many other different brands can find them in the markets.

4. Music: Enjoy your walk while you are listening to the music, however, ensure if you had your earpiece on you while you are walking, to pay attention to your pathway, and the surroundings to avoid any negative consequences, and the same application should be done when it was with a friend.

5. Friends: This outdoor walk can be conducted alone or with a friend.

6. Impact: Walking outdoors are significantly amazing both physically, and psychologically.

7. Treadmills: These are large stationaries machines are usually used for indoor exercises such as running, climbing, and walking exercises, while they are placed in same place, and they comes in different designs, and brands, and sometimes can be placed outside, and operated outside too, and this is depend on the personal preferences, because some people prefer to exercise on treadmill while they are outside, and if you are one of those people and you are already familiar with it, and you are planning to use it for

walking, then that's great, however ensure to adjust the treadmill according to your walking objectives, and also to follow the safety instructions on it, but if you are not familiar with it, and you are planning to use it outside, then ensure to have somebody familiar with it, to explain to you the details of how to be operated and the functions of everything in it, and the safety instructions too, and not just that, conduct the exercise under direct supervision until you become familiar with it, and after that, everything is on your own and lastly, remember that treadmill is for individual use only, and outcomes from using it, are great too.

INDOOR SAFETY PROCEDURES:

These applies when you are planning to conduct the walk indoor such as in a Physical Fitness Facility or any Sports Indoor buildings or inside a home, and so on, and most of the time, walking indoor conducted on the treadmill, and these indoor safety procedures as follows:

1. Pathways: If you are planning to walk inside a building used for sports activities other than a physical

fitness facility such as the Gym, ensure to know your pathway, to prevent injuries, and be considerate, and respectful to others if there are any.

2. Affordable Attire: Wear the proper clothes (top, bottom, footwear, and a sleeve if you are in need for it such as knee sleeves, calf sleeves, and so on), that will suit your walking and make you comfortable while inside, and it gives you the support, and protection.

3. Music: Enjoy your indoor walk while you are listening to the music, however, ensure if you had your earpiece on you while you are walking, to pay attention to your pathway, and to the surroundings, and the same application should be done when it was with a friend.

4. Friends: The indoor walking can be conducted alone or with a friend.

5. Impact: Walking indoors are significantly amazing both physically, and psychologically, however

walking outdoors are more significantly amazing when it comes to the psychological impact.

6. Treadmill: As it was stated earlier in the outdoor safety procedures that treadmills are mostly used for indoor running, climbing, and walking exercises so if you are one of those people who likes to conduct the walking exercise on treadmill, and you are already familiar with it then that's great, however er ensure to adjust the treadmill according to your walking objectives, and also to follow the safety instructions on it, but if you are not familiar with it, and you would like to utilized for first time then ensure to have somebody familiar with it, to explain to you the details of how to operated and the functions of everything in it, and the safety instructions too, and not just that, conduct the exercise under direct supervision until you become familiar with it, and after that, everything is on your own, and lastly, remember that treadmill is for individual use only, and outcomes from using it, are significantly great.

TYPES EXPLANATION

1-SHORT WALK EXERCISE:

This exercise is for the ones who's never done any exercise, and plans to do the walking exercise or for somebody has been doing it but not very constantly, or for a senior people or people with some medical conditions that does not prevent them from doing it, therefore the short walk exercise is their best option, with either own pace or whatever comfortable pace they feel to do it, **and this short walk can be done for 20-30 minutes** however **depending on the person's age, physical capability, and health conditions**, the duration of this short walk can be **adjusted to 10-15 minutes**, and this can be apply for senior people or people with some medical conditions.

As far as how frequently this walk can be done in a week, and the answer to that, is that this exercise can be done **in every day or every other day**, and nothing wrong with that, but **recovery** is very important, and also sometimes **doing the same exercise in every single day, it might become boring for some people or sometimes some people cannot do it in every single day due to their life responsibilities, so time balancing between life responsibilities, and the exercise are very important** too, therefore it is very important to take all these considerations in the mind, and personally, I believed doing the exercise in every other day is very necessary, and important for us, and that is **for two reasons**, and the first reason which is to allow our bodies to have enough time for recovery, and to replenish whatever nutrition was lost from exercising, and the second reason, which is to allow us to balance our time between the exercise and taking care of our life daily responsibilities while we resting from the exercise.

Moreover short walk exercise has a lot of health benefits for the body in both aspects physically and mentally, and if you continue doing only the short walk as your walking exercise, then that's a great, however if you are feeling comfortable about progressing your short walk exercise to the second type of Homeless People Exercise (HPE) which is the Long Walk, then that is significantly amazing too.

2-LONG WALK EXERCISE:

This is for people whose been already done the short walk exercise, and their bodies have been built the strength to do the long walk, and they are feeling comfortable to do it, therefore long walk exercise is their best option, and **this long walk can be done from 30-45 mins, and above**, while the pace can be either own pace or whatever comfortable pace or can be advance into a faster pace, since the ones , whose doing it, were already experienced the short walk, however **depending on the person's age, physical capability, and health conditions**, the duration of this long walk exercise can **be adjusted to 20-30 minutes**, and this can be apply for senior people or people with some medical conditions.

As far as the how frequently this exercise can be done, it should be similar to the short walk exercise however with taken in the considerations the time for recovery, and to avoid from making the exercise boring, and lastly to create a time balance between the exercise, and daily life responsibilities.

NUTRITION

Generally, nutrition, and eating regularly are very important, and necessary supplements for our bodies, because they provide the energy, and support that our bodies needs to develop, and to function properly on daily basis, and to protect us from diseases, and to replenish, and balance whatever our bodies loss from vitamins, and minerals during practicing our daily life routine, and lack of these nutrition, could lead to plenty of health risk factors, and remember consuming a healthy nutrition is vital key for a healthier life condition.

As far as the Homeless People Exercise (HPE), since its goal to target all people from different ages, and different life categories, and we all know for the fact, that nowadays, the market prices as far as the food, water, and other life necessities have been going up, and continue to going up, and not everyone can afford the rising in the prices, and with taken all of that in the considerations, therefore the Homeless People Exercise (HPE) does not require a special or restrict diet or nutrition that needs to follow, and you can eat, and drink whatever you likes to eat, and drink, however there are an important considerations that need to be followed for the health benefits, and to achieve the best results of the Homeless People Exersicse (HPE), and because they are important, I called them **the Red Lines considerations**, and there are four of these Red Lines Considerations, and these four Red Lines consideration as follows:

RED LINE ONE:

Red Line One, means to eat, and drink whatever makes you comfortable, and happy about it, to enjoy your life to the fullest, and to replenish your body from whatever energy lost from doing the Homeless People Exercise, but **ensure, and always remember this, and this is very important to know**, that whatever you eats, and drinks, are not going to cause a negative consequences on your health condition for long run, because the goal here is that we need to stay healthier as much as we can, therefore you need to be considerate about your age, sex, race, ethnicity, gender and background, and carefully watch of what are you consuming.

RED LINE TWO:

Red Line Two means that the status of your health need to be monitored all the time regardless , however if you have any medical conditions, then you have to eats, and drinks whatever suit your medical conditions, and always seeks a consultation from your medical professional about it, and prior to start the exercise, and at the same time, give yourself the nutrition that your body needs to replenish whatever you are lost from exercising the Homeless People Exercise (HPE), to achieve the best results of it, and maintaining your healthiness.

RED LINE THREE:

Red Line Three means that you need to stay hydrated at all the times regardless, and drinking water is the best way of it. Since the Homeless People Exercise (HPE) is a physical activity that will lead to fluids loss, therefore it is very important to maintain your level of hydration perfectly to achieve the best the of it, and I do not want to make it complicated and confusion to you, by telling you how much amounts of fluids or water that you need to take per day, and instead of that, I need you to use your common sense, and drink whatever make you feel that your body is well hydrated, and ready for the Homeless People Exercise (HPE), however you need to remember an important thing which is not to over-hydrated or dehydrated because the two of them could lead to a health issues in the body, and if you were practicing the exercise in hot weather ensure to have enough hydration to replenish whatever you are going to lose during the exercise.

RED LINE FOUR:

Walking has a great health benefit on the body, despite to that, if you are planning to execute the Homeless People Exercise (HPE), and prior to do that, ensure, and always to seek a medical consultation with your medical professional to ensure that you are eligible to do that to avoid any medical complications later on.

RECOVERY

If you want to be a doctor or lawyer you have to study hard for it, and it will require you certain hours a day for example 5-6 hours at least, however you cannot study all these 5-6hours without having a breaks in between, because your mind will be tired, and you will have a difficulty to store and retrieve any study materials from you mind, and if you continue doing that constantly and for a period of time, then your mind will be burnt, and your studying will be a waste of time, and efforts, and you will not be able to reach your goal whether to be a doctor or a lawyer, despite to that, if you planned to take breaks very frequently during your hard study, then you are given your mind the opportunity to rest and refresh and the longevity to store and retrieve your study materials and by doing that, it will help you to reach your goal which is to become a doctor or lawyer, and this is apply too, if you want to be a boxer or a soccer player or any other career fields, and you have to work, and train hard for it for certain hours a day, however you cannot work or train hard all day long without having breaks, because your body will be tired both mentally, and physically, and you won't be able to reach your goal which is to become a boxer or a soccer player, and the points from these examples, are showing that having a frequent and constant breaks from anything we do in life, is very healthy, and everyone should work with it.

Basically, the concept of having **a break frequently, and constantly** is applies **to broader aspects and fields in our life**, and it is very important, because as a human, it will give us the opportunity to rest both mentally, and physically, and doing that, it will help us to reassess our thoughts, and focus on our goals.

In terms of sports, recovery is very important, and this concept of having breaks frequently, and constantly have been always taken in the considerations for any type of sports, whether on the sports level itself or the players levels and it is one of the important factors to achieve the best results for the sport itself, and the players too.

You can practice or exercise any type of sports for a day or a week or a month and even a year, As long as you taken enough time for **recovery**, then you are good, because recovery will give the body the time to rest, and the longevity to continue with whatever sport you are practicing or exercising, and there is nothing wrong whether you practice or exercise for 6 days a week and 1 day off for recovery or whatever your training schedule is as long as you ensure there is a time for recovery included in it.

As far as **the Homeless People Exercise Recovery (HPE)**, and as it was stated earlier, it targeted people from all ages, with different life categories, and the goal from doing it, is to stay in healthier condition, it is recommended to conducted the exercise every other day, and there are two reason behind that, the first reason which is to allow our bodies to have enough time for recovery, and to replenish whatever nutrition lost from exercising, and the second reason, which is to allow us to balance our time between the exercise, and taking care of our life daily responsibilities while we resting from the exercise.

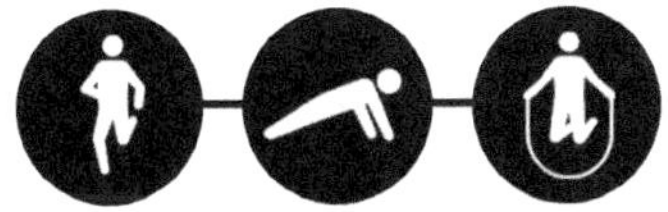

PROS, AND CONS

PROS:

1. Mental impact: Great way for relaxation from what we through in daily basis and boost the motivation and refresh the mind.

2. Physical impact: Doing exercise regularly helps in keeping the body in fine shape.

3. Medical impact: Doing exercise regularly has plenty of positive impact on the body such as improving, and strength the health of the heart, lowering the blood pressure, lowering blood sugar, sedated joints pain, and so many others.

4. Strength Immunity: Doing exercise regularly, strength the health of your immune system, and helps in preventing and controlling diseases.

5. Weight loss: Doing exercise regularly helps to burn calories that lead to losing weight.

6. Healthy body: Doing exercise regularly will help to maintain a healthier body.

7. Socializing: Doing exercise regularly is a great opportunity to socialize with others for fun, however it can be done alone or with friends.

8. Multiple health benefits: Doing exercise regularly has plenty of health benefits, more than the one mentioned above, because the exercise is very powerful, therefore it is recommended to continue doing the exercise regularly.

CONS:

1. Overwalking: It is true that walking is very low impact exercise with very little risk involved despite to that, doing the exercise more than the supposed to, it might increase that risk.

2. Impact:
   A. Mental Impact: doing the exercise in every single day is a great, however this might be become boring for some people whose busy with life, and other challenges, and for that reason, and as it was stated earlier, doing the exercise in every other day, it is recommended to have the people the time to balance between their life, and the exercise, and the most important to have a time for recovery.

   B. Physical impact: doing exercise every single day is great too, however it might increase the risk of having soreness, and muscle fatigue in the body particularly the lower part, therefore doing the exercise in every other day, it is recommended to avoid all of that.

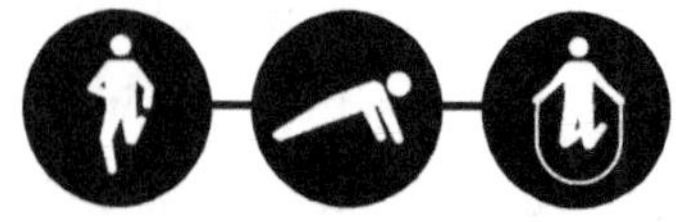

CONCLUSION

Life and death is a God matter, and we as human we have no control over it, however we have the mankind ability that would help us to be a healthier and lives longer so that we can enjoy the life to the fullest, and to reach all the goals in life, and there are plenty of ways to do that, and applying, practicing, and maintaining a healthy life style is one of these ways that will help us to live longer, and to reach all our goals.

A Healthy lifestyle, is accumulation of many of good healthy things that we need to apply into our life, and practicing and exercising regularly is one of these good healthy things, and Homeless People Exercise (HPE), is a good example of that, and conducting the exercise regularly, it will help us to reach to this healthy life style, and not just that, a Homeless People exercise (HPE), It is one of the most effective and efficient way of exercising that doesn't require any equipment and it can be achieve by anybody at any given time, and place, and if we cannot do the exercise regularly due to some life responsibilities or some difficulties, and that's fine, however ensure to do it at your convenient time, and never ignored it, because the point here, is to do our best be a healthy, and live longer, and for any reasons, that will prevent us from having the opportunity to do the Homeless People Exercise (HPE) nor we cannot exercising at all, then ensure to keep yourself in the move, in other word keeps your body active, because keeping the body physically active, it's another way of exercising that will help us keeps the body healthy.

This booklet is intended for the informational purposes and whatever was in it, was expressed solely by the author personal knowledge, and experience to share it with the public, however the public have the right of the option whether to use it or not, and most importantly and for the confirmation, this booklet, is not intended to provide any type of medical treatment and medical consultation nor to replace any type of medical treatment and medical consultation, and always seeks a consultation with your medical professional or somebody professional in the filed prior to conduct the exercise.

Lastly, my highest gratitude, and tremendous respect to all my readers, and to every living in our world, and remember to stay healthy because life is great.

www.ingramcontent.com/pod-product-compliance
Lightning Source LLC
Chambersburg PA
CBHW052223150726

48002CB00003B/1247